BEEF JERKY FOR WEIGHT LOSS

simply the best jerky you can make, one recipe. The secret.

Adam D. Sanchez

Table of Contents

CHAPTER 1......................5

Is Beef Jerky Healthy for Weight Loss?.........................5

What is beef jerky 7

What are the components of beef jerky.............................18

Does beef jerky make you put on weight..............................21

Is jerky a healthy and balanced treat.......................................23

CHAPTER 2 29

Is Beef Jerky Great for You?.29

Downsides of beef jerky........35

The best ways to make beef jerky in the house 39

The profits.............................42

CHAPTER 3 44

5 UNEXPECTED REASONS BEEF JERKY FOR WEIGHT LOSS IS REAL 44

Lower Line 50

CHAPTER 1

Is Beef Jerky Healthy for Weight Loss?

If you want to know the wellness advantages of beef jerky, you need to make it through all the information concerning it. You're possibly questioning "is beef jerky healthy and balanced for weight-loss?" Discover the solutions in this message.

Beef jerky is an excellent resource of healthy protein, iron, salt, and also several various other dietary variables. You need to preserve the usage quantity and also that is how you can possibly do helpful for your body. Beef jerky has a number of great advantages and also some adverse effects too. In this short post, we are most likely to speak about all these points.

Let's have a look at the information to recognize more concerning it.

What is beef jerky

Beef jerky is refined beef. In the 1800s, it stemmed in Southern The u.s.a.. Nonetheless, different more tastes have been included in it recently to build it flexible.

It's reduced into slim strips and also marinated in a treating salt service. Then, the strips are hung on prepare. It's prepared for about 2.5 to 5 hrs inning accordance with how individuals desire it to be. Keeping all these actions, permits the jerky to be kept for a very long time.

What are the needs to reduce weight if you have actually beef jerky

There are some reasons that beef jerky excels to reduce weight. You can possibly have a great deal of nourishing aspects that aid to build you healthy and balanced and also you will certainly really feel light. Let's see what the nourishing aspects are and also how it aids to reduce weight.

Healthy protein in Weight Loss:

Beef jerky is high in healthy protein. Consuming it has a great deal of wellness advantages. Healthy protein aids to reduce weight. Taking in beef jerky is a means you can possibly pick. It decreases cravings and also cravings and also boosts muscle mass mass, toughness, and also metabolic process.

Besides, healthy protein digests slower compared to carbs. So, you will certainly really feel much less starving. Beef jerky is an advantage due to the fact that it does not generate insulin. So, it can't keep fat. Total, beef jerky can possibly be an excellent service to reducing weight. So, if you have actually an inquiry in your mind, "is beef jerky an excellent resource of healthy protein?", the solution is of course.

Dietary Aspects Aids More:

Beef jerky has different type of dietary components. The dietary variables rely on the brand name. For that, you have to inspect the beef jerky nourishment tag. One ounce of jerky consists of 9 grams of healthy protein, 7 grams of fat, 116 calories, and also 3 grams of carbs. 11% phosphorus, 8% iron, and also 15% everyday worth for immune assistance zinc.

All these points aid to carry oxygen into the body. That improves the beef jerky wellness advantages. The various other point is that it comes in handy and also an excellent resource of healthy protein. It ends up being a general great component making a healthy and balanced dish.

High Quantities of Iron Is Helpful for Weight Loss:

Beef jerky additionally has an excellent quantity of iron. It consists of 1.8 milligrams of iron while ladies call for a minimum of 18 milligrams and also guys call for 8 milligrams of iron each day. Iron is a necessary component for the body. If your body does not have sufficient oxygen, it triggers exhaustion. So, iron aids a great deal in this instance as it can possibly bring oxygen for a body.

Reduced Carbohydrate As Well:

Beef jerky additionally consists of low-carbohydrates centers. This is practical for you to reduce weight. Low-carb foods aid individuals to reduce weight much faster compared to anything else. So, beef jerky may help you with that said. You can possibly utilize beef jerky in a number of diet regimen strategies like Keto, Atkins,

Carnivore diet regimen, Paleo diet regimen, and also more.

Not simply that, it can possibly additionally offer you a great deal of healthy protein and also some fat with no carbs included in it. So, it will certainly be an excellent choice to obtain beef jerky to consist of in your diet regimen strategy. Make certain you obtain the jerky that has no included sugar.

Beef Jerky Is Practical:

Another essential point is comfort. If you can't preserve the diet regimen strategy appropriately, you can't reduce weight. Yet beef jerky followers make you cover. This is the handiest and also a lot of comfy component you can possibly have for your diet regimen. It's very easy to consume as you do not have to prepare it. Additionally, it consists of a great deal of healthy protein that fulfills your body's needs. Pick the most effective sampling beef jerky and also alternating it with your convenience food.

Very easy to Obtain Treat:

Beef jerky is an excellent

choice

if you do not seem like food preparation anything to consume. This is a best treat you can possibly have that additionally aids to reduce weight. It has nourishing aspects that can possibly make you joyful and also boost your task. This can possibly additionally boost metabolic process and also maintain you far from sensation starving.

This is the excellent treat you can possibly consume on the move. It's healthy and balanced, mobile, and also light yet maintains your belly complete too. A lot of notably, it preferences scrumptious. You can possibly additionally obtain self-made beef jerky calories that preference great too. So, if you have actually this beef jerky, you can possibly experience just great points.

You could possibly additionally like: Is Mac and also Cheese Healthy and balanced?

What are the components of beef jerky
beef jerky helpful for you

To learn about the components of beef jerky, you have to inspect the information that we are most likely to reveal you. Let's dive into the information to obtain the total details.

Just what does it cost? healthy protein in beef jerky:

Beef jerky has about 33 grams of healthy protein each 100 grams. Beef jerky is made by drying out it with seasonings and also salt. The meat sheds a great deal of sprinkle throughout the drying out procedure and also the healthy protein obtains condensed.

So, the quantity of healthy protein obtains greater as compared to typical meat. This is how beef jerky ends up being a power-packed healthy protein.

Self-made beef jerky is additionally great and also has different sorts of healthy protein. Is self-made beef jerky helpful for you? You can possibly locate the solution right below.

Does beef jerky have iron:

If you wish to know concerning the iron web content in beef jerky, you will certainly be surprised to recognize that beef jerky is high in zinc and also iron. Because of this, it ends up being an excellent resource of blood cell manufacturing. Due to having actually iron, it can possibly additionally generate zinc that can possibly assistance the body immune system of your body.

If you desire an excellent quantity of iron, you can possibly obtain it from beef jerky. Besides, iron aids to bring oxygen to all the cells of your body. This is how it works to shed fat and also reduce weight too.

Does beef jerky make you put on weight

is beef jerky healthy and balanced for weight-loss

If you question in your mind, "does beef jerky make you fat?" Or "is beef jerky fattening?", you need to learn about beef jerky thoroughly. Although beef jerky has a great deal of great components that are practical to reduce weight, it can possibly additionally be a factor to put on weight if you do not take it appropriately.

Besides, if you consume excessive beef jerky, it avoids you from consuming various other foods. So, you will certainly absence a great deal of various other nutrients that you can't obtain from beef jerky.

Additionally, the calories in beef jerky teriyaki are high. If you eat a great deal of these points, there's a substantial opportunity to put on weight.

Is jerky a healthy and balanced treat

If you have actually an inquiry in your mind, "is beef jerky a healthy and balanced treat?", you have to experience its dietary variables and also the amount that you require. Beef jerky is total a best healthy and balanced treat that you could have at any time you really feel starving.

As it's an excellent resource of healthy protein, iron, and also salt, you can possibly meet your body's needs. So, you can possibly phone telephone call beef jerky a healthy and balanced treat.

Is beef jerky healthy and balanced for weight-loss

is beef jerky fattening

Beef jerky is an excellent resource of different great components. You can possibly have a great deal of advantages with it. There are different type of dietary advantages you can possibly need to reducing weight. Vitamin B12, iron, healthy protein, and also great deals more materials that you have to moisturize your body. All things assistance your body to provide a good quantity of oxygen. And also that is how you can possibly reduce weight properly. Is beef jerky healthy and balanced? Certainly, it's.

Is beef jerky poor

Beef jerky has an excellent quantity of dietary aspects that offer you audio wellness. Yet it additionally has some disadvantages if you eat it in a substantial quantity. If you eat way too much beef jerky, there's an opportunity you deal with a number of illness. This can possibly be a factor for boosting high blood pressure, stroke, and also kidney concerns.

In addition, it can possibly boost cholesterol degrees if you consume excessive beef jerky. If you consume beef jerky, you do not seem like consuming anything greater than that. So, you will certainly be losing out on a great deal more nutrients like fiber, vitamins, and also unsaturated fats that vegetables and fruits can possibly offer you. Obtain beef jerky specific packs so that you could obtain a suggestion concerning just what does it cost? you need to consume.

CHAPTER 2

Is Beef Jerky Great for You?
Beef jerky is a preferred and also hassle-free treat food.

Its name originates from the Quechua word "ch'arki," which means dried, salted meat.

Beef jerky is made from lean reduces of beef that are marinated with different sauces, seasonings, and also various other ingredients. It after that undertakes different refining approaches, such as healing, cigarette smoking cigarettes, and also drying out, previously its packaged available up available.

Due to the fact that jerky is thought about a treat food, many individuals marvel whether it is a healthy and balanced or harmful

choice

.

This short post assesses whether beef jerky benefits you.

Nutrition and potential benefits

Normally talking, beef jerky is a healthy and balanced and also healthy treat.

One ounce (28 grams) of beef jerky consists of the adhering to nutrients:

Calories: 116

Healthy protein: 9.4 grams

Fat: 7.3 grams

Carbohydrates: 3.1 grams

Fiber: 0.5 grams

Zinc: 21% of the Everyday Worth (DV)

Vitamin B12: 12 % of the DV

Phosphorus: 9% of the DV

Folate: 9% of the DV

Iron: 8% of the DV

Copper: 7% of the DV

Choline: 6% of the DV

Selenium: 5% of the DV

Potassium: 4% of the DV

Thiamine: 4% of the DV

Magnesium: 3% of the DV

Riboflavin: 3% of the DV

Niacin: 3% of the DV

It likewise supplies little quantities of manganese, molybdenum, and also pantothenic acid.

Considered that it is high in healthy protein and also reduced in carbohydrates, it has a much healthier dietary make-up compared to lots of various other treat foods and also appropriates for different diet plans, such as reduced carbohydrate and also paleo diet plans.

It is likewise high in different minerals, consisting of zinc and also iron, which are essential for lots of works, consisting of immune and also power degree assistance.

What is more, beef jerky has a lengthy service life and also is extremely mobile, that makes it a wonderful choice for take a trip, backpacking, and also various other circumstances where you have restricted accessibility to fresh food and also require a healthy protein strike.

SUMMARY

Beef jerky is a great resource of healthy protein and also high in lots of minerals and vitamins, consisting of zinc, iron, vitamin B12, phosphorus, and also folate. It likewise has a lengthy service life and also is mobile, production it a wonderful on-the-go choice.

Downsides of beef jerky
However beef jerky is a nourishing treat, it must be eaten in small amounts.

It is extremely high in salt, with a 1-ounce (28-gram) offering supplying approximately 22% of your everyday salt allocation, which is evaluated 2,300 mg daily.

Extreme salt consumption could damage numerous elements of your health and wellness, consisting of heart health and wellness, high blood pressure, and also stroke threat.

That likewise makes it unsuitable for sure diet plans that limit salt consumption.

Additionally, beef jerky is very refined. Various research researches have revealed a link in between diet plans high in refined and also healed red meats like beef jerky and also a greater threat of cancers cells, such as intestinal cancers cells.

Furthermore, a current examine discovered that dried out, healed meats like beef jerky could be infected with harmful materials called mycotoxins, which are created by fungis that expand on meat. Study has connected mycotoxins to cancer cells.

Simply put, however beef jerky is a healthy and balanced treat, its ideal eaten in small amounts. A lot of your diet regimen must originate from entire, unprocessed foods.

SUMMARY

However beef jerky is healthy and balanced, prevent consuming way too much of it, as it is high in salt and also could feature the exact same health and wellness dangers that are

connected to consuming refined
meats.

The best ways to make beef jerky in the house

It is simple to create your very
own beef jerky in the house.

Doing so is likewise an excellent
way to regulate all the active
ingredients, particularly salt.

To create beef jerky in the house,
merely utilize a lean reduced of
beef, such as leading rounded,
eye of rounded, lower rounded,

sirloin idea, or flank steak, and also piece the beef into slim pieces.

After cutting, marinade the meat in natural herbs, seasonings, and also sauces of your selection. Later, rub the jerky strips completely dry to eliminate any kind of extra marinade and also area them in a meat dehydrator at 155-165°F (68-74°C) for roughly 4-5 hrs — depending upon the meat's density.

If you do not have a dehydrator, you can possibly attain comparable outcomes utilizing a stove at a reduced temperature level — roughly 140-170°F (60-75°C) for 4-5 hrs.

What is more, it is a great idea to allow the beef jerky dehydrate additional at space temperature level for an added 24 hr previously you plan it. It could be ideal to ice up jerky if you're not most likely to consume it within 1 week approximately.

SUMMARY

Beef jerky is straightforward to create in the house and also enables you to regulate all the active ingredients, especially salt.

The profits

Beef jerky is a wonderful treat food that is high in healthy protein and also a great resource of different minerals, consisting of zinc and also iron.

Nevertheless, store-bought selections are high in salt and

also could be connected with various other dangers, so it is ideal eaten in small amounts as section of a different diet regimen.

That stated, production your very own jerky is straightforward and also can possibly aid regulate its salt material.

CHAPTER 3

5 UNEXPECTED REASONS BEEF JERKY FOR WEIGHT LOSS IS REAL

Beef jerky can possibly be a tasty and also efficient section of a healthy and balanced diet regimen for weight management. It's a functional and also hassle-free treat that may help you not just drop weight yet likewise maintain it off.

Right below are 5 reasons beef jerky can possibly assist with weight management and also living a healthy and balanced way of life.

Beef Jerky on white history.

1. Nutrition Thick

Beef jerky was a diet regimen staple for healthy and balanced individuals for centuries. The primary factor? It's nutrition thick. The proportion of calories to nutrients is off the graphes. It can possibly supply as much as 15g of healthy protein each 100 calories. That suggests no vacant calories. Your calories are functioning as difficult as you when you treat on beef jerky.

2. Loaded with Healthy protein

The primary component in beef jerky is beef, which is normally high in healthy protein. Consuming a diet regimen abundant in healthy protein has lots of health and wellness advantages relates to weight management. Eating healthy protein can possibly minimize hunger and also appetite, raise stamina and also muscular tissue mass, and also rev up your metabolic rate. When you are sensation starving, grab beef jerky to obtain healthy protein that will maintain you sustained.

3. Iron Abundant

Beef jerky supplies a healthy and balanced dosage of iron, an essential and also under-appreciated mineral. Iron aids bring oxygen to all cells in your body, consisting of muscular tissues. This aids melt fat.

Iron shortage can possibly reduce power sources and also make workout challenging. A healthy and balanced diet regimen abundant in iron can possibly maintain you sustained and also invigorated and also all set to take on workout.

4. Hassle-free

Lots of weight management initiatives go off the rails when active lives hinder. Beef jerky is hassle-free, mobile, and also does not need any kind of food preparation. It provides healthy protein on-the-go. You can possibly load beef jerky in the car so when a desire for processed food strikes, you can possibly grab a healthy and balanced treat choice.

5. Excellent for Any kind of Reduced Carbohydrate Diet regimen

There's expanding proof that a low-carbohydrate diet regimen aids individuals drop weight quicker and also efficiently compared to a low-fat diet regimen. There's likewise expanding proof that it aids individuals keep weight management.

There are lots of variants of a low-carb diet—Keto diet regimen, Carnivore Diet regimen, Atkins, Paleo Diet regimen. No matter your choice, beef jerky can possibly supply healthy protein and also fat with no included carbs. See to it to acquire beef jerky that has no included sugar.

Lower Line

Many individuals wonder—is beef jerky healthy and balanced? When eaten as section of a well-rounded diet regimen, it can possibly definitely aid in dropping weight. The vital is picking the appropriate beef jerky.

With absolutely no sugar and also no synthetic active ingredients, our beef jerky is the very best beef jerky for weight management. See to it to pick the choices that are sugar-free.